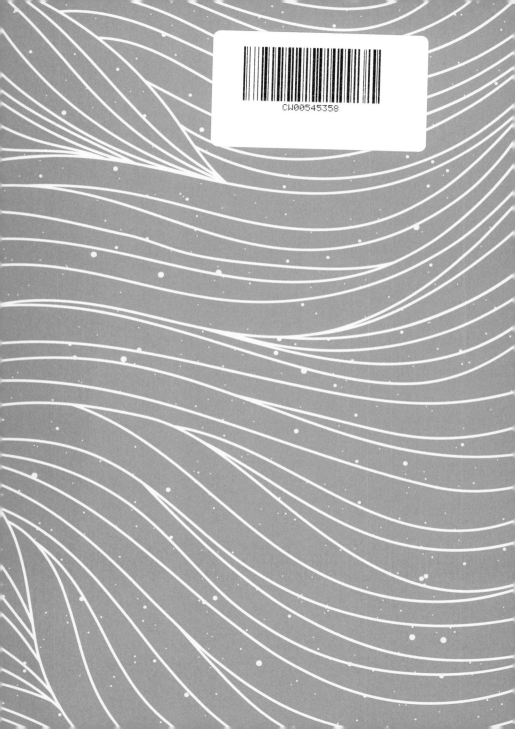

FIND
YOUR
FLOW

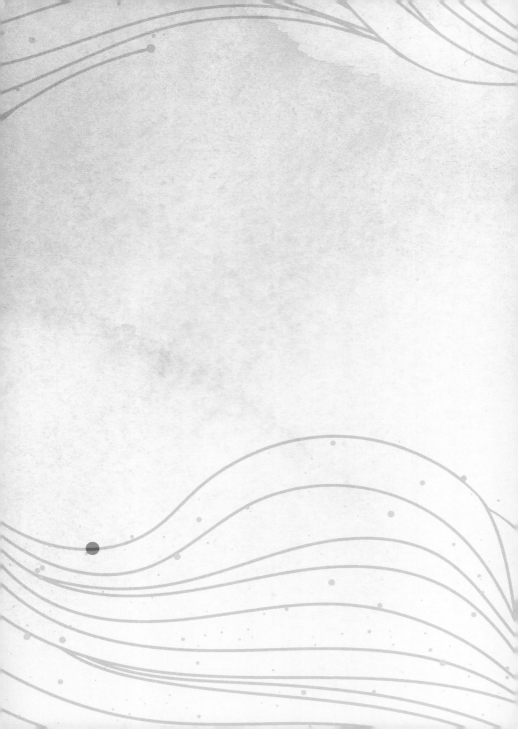

FIND YOUR FLOW

THE SIMPLE AND LIFE-CHANGING PRACTICE FOR A HAPPIER YOU

SARAH GREGG

ROCK
POINT

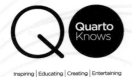

Inspiring | Educating | Creating | Entertaining

Brimming with creative inspiration, how-to projects, and useful information to enrich your everyday life, Quarto Knows is a favorite destination for those pursuing their interests and passions. Visit our site and dig deeper with our books into your area of interest: Quarto Creates, Quarto Cooks, Quarto Homes, Quarto Lives, Quarto Drives, Quarto Explores, Quarto Gifts, or Quarto Kids.

Text © 2020 Sarah Gregg
Cover art © Yellena James

First published in 2020 by Rock Point, an imprint of The Quarto Group,
142 West 36th Street, 4th Floor, New York, NY 10018, USA
T (212) 779-4972 F (212) 779-6058 www.QuartoKnows.com

Rock Point titles are also available at discount for retail, wholesale, promotional and bulk purchase. For details, contact the Special Sales Manager by email at specialsales@quarto.com or by mail at The Quarto Group, Attn: Special Sales Manager, 100 Cummings Center Suite, 265D, Beverly, MA 01915, USA.

10 9 8 7 6 5 4 3 2 1

ISBN: 978-1-63106-629-0

Library of Congress Cataloging-in-Publication Data

Names: Gregg, Sarah, author.
Title: Find your flow : the simple and life-changing practice for a happier you /
    Sarah Gregg.
Description: New York, NY : Rock Point, 2020. | Includes bibliographical
    references and index. | Summary: "Discover your ideal state of happiness
    with the powerful yet simple practices set forth in Find Your Flow"--
    Provided by publisher.
Identifiers: LCCN 2019034972 (print) | LCCN 2019034973 (ebook) | ISBN
    9781631066290 (hardcover) | ISBN 9780760365601 (ebook)
Subjects: LCSH: Self-actualization (Psychology) | Self-realization. |
    Change (Psychology)
Classification: LCC BF637.S4 G743 2020 (print) | LCC BF637.S4 (ebook) |
    DDC 158.1--dc23
LC record available at https://lccn.loc.gov/2019034972
LC ebook record available at https://lccn.loc.gov/2019034973

Publisher: Rage Kindelsperger
Creative Director: Laura Drew
Managing Editor: Cara Donaldson
Senior Editor: Erin Canning
Art Director: Cindy Samargia Laun
Cover and Interior Design: Jen Cogliantry
Author Photograph: Kyle Brereton

Printed in China

To all those
brave enough
to become
who they truly are,
stay courageous.

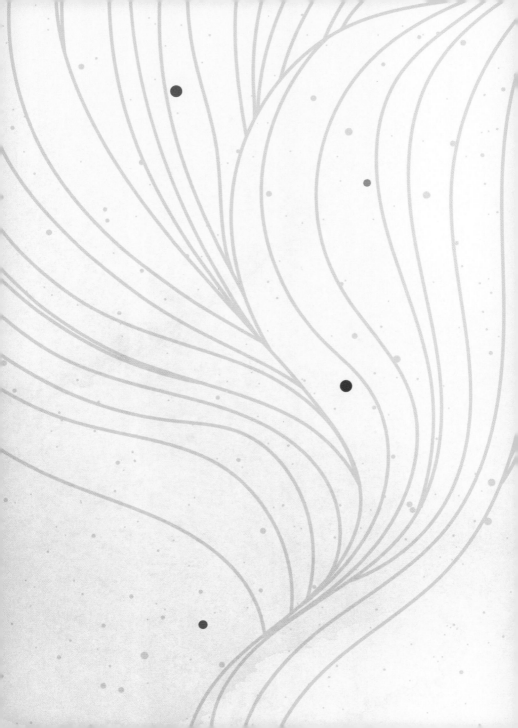

CONTENTS

Those who
flow
as life flows
know
They need no
other force.

— LAO TZU

PREFACE

I've always wanted to live life to the fullest—do as much as I can with the gift of life without wasting my time or potential. And yet, despite these intentions, I somehow ended up living in a world where I felt overwhelmed and frustrated by life. I was thirty-four and had worked hard to climb the career ladder. I had a great job as a business advisor at a local university, lived in a nice house with my husband, Chris, and drove a good car. For all intents and purposes, my life on the outside seemed "normal," so why did I feel unhappy and lost?

On my journey to find the root of my discontent, I realized happiness eluded me because I had attached it to success. I would tell myself that I could relax, be happy, and enjoy life only when I achieved this or gained that. I believed that in order to feel worthy of happiness, everything needed to be "perfect." And as a result, I was locked in a never-ending cycle of chasing this "perfection." My overreliance on the outside world to provide me with happiness through achievements, accolades, praise, status, and the feeling of superiority had disconnected me from my ability to cultivate happiness.

I was filled with self-doubt, self-sabotage, self-comparison, fear, worry, and feelings of inadequacy. I compared myself to others and became resentful of their happiness. And what made the process even harder was my inability to tell friends because of the shame and guilt I was feeling. I tried to outrun my uncomfortable feelings with distractions and a busy schedule. But in the months leading up to my thirty-fourth birthday, I became exhausted and feared that if I continued to run away from these problems, I would eventually burn out.

My life felt out of control and alignment and lacked meaning and direction. But at the same time, there was the light of "knowing" that there was more to life than I was currently experiencing, a hopeful energy that pulled me to explore a world beyond feeling just "fine." I knew I had to change, take responsibility, and regain control of my life. I wanted to find a way of living that balanced my everyday happiness with my future ambitions.

Some people think the turning point in my life was when my husband and I sold our house and all our belongings to set up our own businesses and pursue our dreams of combining work and travel. But they are wrong. What really changed my experience of life (inside and out) was discovering the surprising psychology of flow and the secrets it held to living a happy life.

It was psychologist Mihaly Csikszentmihalyi who first identified and named the psychological concept of "flow," hailing it as the "secret to happiness" in his 2004 TED talk.[1] Flow is a state you can control, create, and experience every day. When in flow, you are able to bring intention, energy, and skills to the present moment that not only bring everyday happiness, but also influence the future and help fulfill your potential.

You may have picked up this book because you want to improve certain areas of your life. Or perhaps you also feel that deep sense of "knowing" that life can be so much more. Perhaps you've found yourself treating life as a problem to be solved, rather than a gift to be experienced. Maybe you're tired of being stuck in a cycle of unhelpful habits. Or maybe you feel unfulfilled because no matter what you do or how much you have, it never feels like enough. Do you want to feel the harmony of alignment as you consistently focus on what matters most each day? Would you like to fulfill your potential and make your signature impact on the world? And if so, have you opened this book seeking guidance on how finding your flow can help create this change?

BUT HOW CAN YOU FIND YOUR FLOW?

This simple question marked the start of my year-and-a-half-long journey to finding flow. Through this process of self-discovery, I created a journal system for flow based on positive psychology that is meant to be used every day. At first, this system for flow was intended for my personal use, but as I saw it transform my own life, I realized I had to share it with others. Then as I watched the life-changing impact it had on my family and friends, I knew that I had to share the secret of flow with the world. And so here we are.

Whatever brought you here, I am grateful that the universe conspired to bring this book to you. I'm honored to guide you on your own, unique journey to finding your flow. This book is written with love, expertise, passion, and vulnerability so that you can fully experience life starting today. It is designed to be practical and actionable. Here's what you can expect on your journey to find your flow:

- A four-step journal system based on the positive psychology of flow that can be instantly applied to your everyday life. All you need to do is invest a few minutes first thing in the morning and again before bed.

- Easy-to-implement, psychology-based tactics that will help you wake up feeling happier, focus on what's important, and defend yourself from distraction so you can get the most out of every day. You will also learn how to lean into life lessons so that you can break unhelpful habits and challenge your limiting beliefs.

- Discovery of the science behind how to create the happiness and serenity that come from flow.

- A journal system that embraces your uniqueness and ditches the "one-size-fits-all" approach to how you should live your life. You'll learn that while the system to find flow may be universal, the flow you will uncover is as unique as you are to the world. This system will awaken and strengthen your authentic voice so that you can make your signature impact on the world, inspire others, and reach your full potential.

The journal system in *Find Your Flow* will help you feel yourself living in alignment and discover there is no need to settle for a life that's mediocre. Today is the day you get out of your own way and experience the happiness you deserve. So, if you're ready to discover the simple yet life-changing journal system to flow, let's not waste any more precious time and begin.

—Sarah Gregg

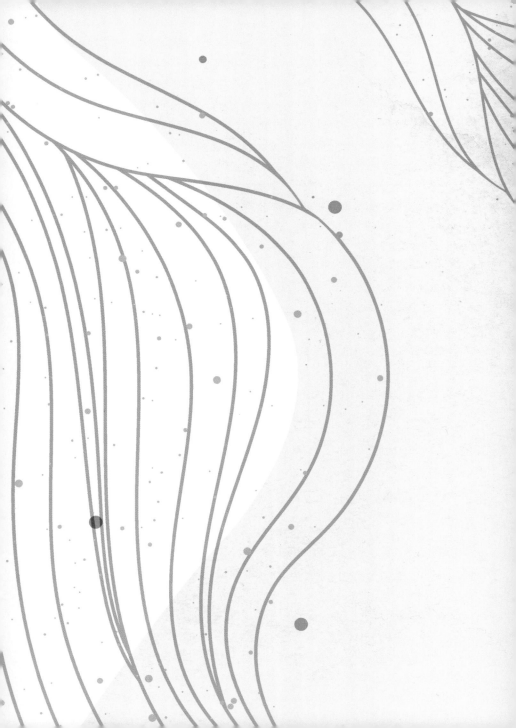

INTRODUCTION:
FLOW AND
HOW TO FIND IT

You feel
Connected
Alive
Aligned
and
Authentically you
As you surrender
To the beautiful imperfect
perfection of life
As it is
And as you do
You notice
How you move with the
natural rhythm of life
Emerged in its current of total
engagement, you
FIND YOUR FLOW

The word flow appears throughout human history, from the ancient Chinese philosopher Lao Tzu, who wrote, "Those who flow as life flows know They need no other force," to modern-day guru Oprah Winfrey, who said, "There is a flow with your name on it. Your job is to find that flow and let it carry you to the next level."

The word flow resonates with us all, but what does it mean? And why is it so important that you find it?

WHAT IS FLOW?

The psychological concept of "flow" was first coined by psychologist and flow expert Mihaly Csikszentmihalyi in the 1970s. He defined flow as an optimal experience and the total involvement in life and found that individuals who experienced flow felt a sense of harmony, serenity, and happiness. Far from "going with the flow," he found that flow was a discipline to bring control and order to your inner life.

In flow, what you wish, think, say, feel, and do align with your goals. It's this feeling of being in congruence with your goals that enables your attention to flow effortlessly into what matters most. For flow to occur, it's important that your goal challenges and stretches your current level of skills. As you invest your energy and skills to overcome that challenge, action and awareness merge, and you become totally absorbed in life. Flow will help you be happy in the present, channel your ambition for the future, and develop your skills so you can fulfill your potential.

It's important to remember that flow is not passively moving in whatever direction life takes you. Flow is taking control and ownership for the direction you want your life to go in. It's this inner order and control that release you of conflicting desires and enable you to fully focus your mental energy on the goals that matter most to you, rather than unnecessarily wasting it on worry, fear, anger, or doubt.

HOW DO YOU EXPERIENCE FLOW?

In his extensive work on flow, Csikszentmihalyi found that we can experience flow in two ways: flow experiences and unified flow.

Flow experiences are brief, exceptional moments of flow. Csikszentmihalyi writes that "flow experiences provide the flashes of intense living."[2] It's in flow experiences that you lose your sense of self, worries disappear, and time slows down. Flow experiences often occur in activities such as playing music, sports, and chess; problem-solving; and even having an interesting conversation with friends. People often describe flow experiences as "being in the zone," and Csikszentmihalyi found these experiences to be important because they add pleasure to the present moment, build confidence, and develop skills. However, flow experiences are short-lived, and although important to identify, when used in isolation, they will not create a life of meaning and purpose.

Csikszentmihalyi describes **unified flow** as when "an important goal is pursued with resolution."[3] The goal must be of personal significance, whether you want to perform on Broadway, raise a family, own a business, or find a solution to climate change. Csikszentmihalyi writes, "If a person sets out to achieve a difficult enough goal, from which all other goals logically follow, and if he or she invests all energy in developing skills to reach that goal, then actions and feelings will be in harmony, and the separate parts of life will fit together. . . . In such a way, it is possible to give meaning to one's entire life."[4] The journal system provides the structure to find both flow experiences and unified flow.

HOW DO YOU
FIND FLOW?

"If we agree that the bottom line of life is happiness, not success, then it makes perfect sense to say that it is the journey that counts, not reaching the destination."

—Mihaly Csikszentmihalyi, *Good Business*

Flow embraces individuality because what creates flow for one person may not create flow for another. The journey to find your flow will be a personal one, and although the system will be the same, what you put into it and how it transforms your life will be unique to you.

Find Your Flow shares the journal system for flow based on positive psychology research and specifically designed to fit busy lives. This book takes the theory of flow and shows you how you can put it into practice—simply and easily—every day. It does more than get you to think differently about your life; it shows you how to apply that thinking by changing your daily practices. The journal system is based upon the research of positive psychology and neuroscience, drawing upon the work of Csikszentmihalyi. The journal system for flow you're about to discover here integrates the three core conditions that Csikszentmihalyi found necessary for flow to occur: clear goals (I know what I am doing and why), optimal level of challenge (I will complete my goal to the best of my current ability so that it stretches my skills), and immediate feedback (I understand what successful progress toward my goal looks, feels, and sounds like). It's these three core conditions, along with feeling positive and reflecting, that I have discovered are important for finding and staying in everyday flow. Over the course of each chapter, you'll dive into the psychology and science of how that specific part of the system will help you find your flow. Here's an overview of the system you will work with.

MORNING GRATEFUL FLOW:
WAKE UP HAPPY

Psychologists have proven that our morning mood can set the tone for the rest of the day, and with Morning Grateful Flow, you'll wake up happy as you start your day writing words of gratitude for the present moment. As feelings of gratitude arise, they will lay the foundations for flow, release inner resistance and create clarity to help you plan the day ahead.

FORWARD FOCUS:
LIVE WITH INTENTION

Forward Focus ensures you live each day with intention. First, you'll spend a few minutes identifying your high-value and high-flow priorities to bring a sense of harmony and balance between what you must do and what you want to do. It's here that you'll see yourself make small, everyday steps to enjoy the present and create your future with intention. You'll learn how to align your intentions and values with your actions and purposefully move toward what matters most.

TOTAL FLOW:
TRAIN YOUR BRAIN

We've all experienced starting the day with good intentions only to spend the rest of the day getting caught up in situations that don't really matter, being easily distracted, or repeating old, unhealthy habits. In Total Flow, you'll spend a few minutes of your morning scripting your ideal day. You'll learn to use imagery scripting, a technique used by elite athletes, to train your attention to spot opportunities, stay on course, and defend yourself against distraction.

NIGHTTIME REFLECTION:
BECOME AWARE, GROW, AND FLOW

Nighttime Reflection is your bedtime journal routine. It's your daily opportunity to lean into the lessons that are showing up in life, spot opportunities to find more flow, and celebrate the powerful small steps you're taking each day to create meaningful life changes.

HOW TO USE
THIS BOOK

The psychology-inspired journal system in *Find Your Flow* is designed to be followed in sequential order, with each practice feeding into the next. So, in order to get maximum value, you should read this book in the order it's presented in. *Find Your Flow* is a journal system that helps you listen to your own inner voice, discover your own answers, and find your unique flow.

At the start of each chapter, I share a story of how my old habits were creating resistance in my life. Then together, we dive into the fascinating psychology of flow, discovering tips and strategies to help you get the most out of the journal system. At the end of each chapter are clear step-by-step instructions on how to practice it.

It's important to remember that although this book teaches you what is possible, it's only through implementation and learning that your potential becomes a reality. For ease of reference, there is a short summary of how the system works along with journal pages starting on page 95 to help you develop a daily practice for finding your flow.

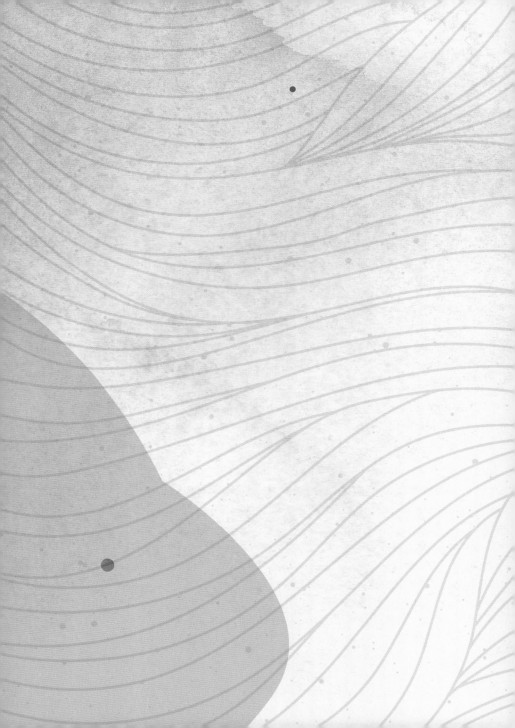

MORNING GRATEFUL FLOW:

WAKE UP HAPPY

Awake
Arise
Absorb
The still beauty
of a new day
And descend
Into its untouched waters
Gently
Gracefully
Writing words
of gratitude with

MORNING
GRATEFUL FLOW

MY OLD
MORNING RITUAL

I reach for my phone on the bedside table. It's Monday morning, and my alarm has gone off. Adjusting my eyes to the light, I turn off the phone alarm and begin my morning ritual of opening apps on my phone. I greet the day by mindlessly scrolling through news articles, social media, and emails. Taking time to read the thoughts of others before considering my own, I flippantly switch from one tab to the next without any intention.

This mindless morning ritual was a direct reflection of my life: always on the go, constantly comparing myself to others, and rarely being fully present to enjoy everything I'd worked so hard to create.

While seemingly innocent, checking my phone first thing in the morning was an unnecessary roll of an emotional die, a naive gamble that could determine the unfolding energy of the day ahead. The information on my phone screen stimulated my brain, sparking a neurological chain reaction of thoughts, feelings, and emotional responses. I used to lie in bed every morning, snuggled in the comfort of my warm duvet, as I rolled the die again and again with app after app. One particular morning, I felt a warmth of positive emotions as I swiped through memories on social media only to feel them quickly replaced by negative emotions when I opened and read a disgruntled email from my manager, Julie.

By the time I sat down to eat breakfast, my negative trickle of thoughts over Julie's email brewed into an almighty storm swirling around my mind. Pouring a coffee, my negative energy overflowed into an ugly, anger-fuelled rant about Julie to my husband, Chris.

I drove impatiently to work, arriving for my 9:00 a.m. meeting frustrated and agitated. Taking my seat at the table, I struggled to focus. I glared vacantly at a report placed in front of me as my mind wandered through various imaginary arguments with Julie. My bad mood had taken over, and its ferocious current carried me through the day.

My negative energy seeped into every crevice of my being, spreading like a virus; I contaminated others with the sour tone of my emails, poisoned colleagues with stories of Julie, and infected those around me with my negativity. After work, I dropped my bags, released a weary sigh, poured a large glass of red wine, and put on the TV to numb my cyclone of emotions. I blamed Julie, my coworkers, and everyone else but myself for my awful day. Yet the following day, I'd gamble with my emotions again, totally oblivious to the impact of my subtle morning ritual.

It wasn't until I began the search to find my flow that my morning ritual of checking my phone was pulled into focus and challenged. I knew from my research that positive emotions facilitated flow, because when we feel good, we can focus and channel our attention onto any given task with greater ease. But it was upon discovering the research about the fragility of our mornings, and the impact it can have on our moods, that I knew my morning habit had to change.

Understanding the importance of my morning mood and its potential to impact my entire day marked the start of my journey to finding flow. And so it's beautifully apt that your journey will also begin with a positive morning ritual.

IT ALL STARTS WITH HOW YOU WAKE UP IN THE MORNING

A study by professor Nancy Rothbard and associate professor Steffanie Wilk found that employees who started the day feeling happy or calm usually stayed in a positive emotional state throughout their workday. However, those who started the day in a bad mood, mostly remained in that mood throughout the day (or even reported feeling *worse* by the end of the day). Furthermore, the study revealed that employees who reported feeling negative emotions took more frequent breaks throughout the day, resulting in more than 10 percent loss of productivity. The researchers concluded that the "start-of-the-day mood can last longer than you might think—and have an important effect on job performance."[5]

I found this study to be fascinating, but the skeptic in me wondered if the results were enough to warrant changing my customary morning app scroll. A study by Harvard researcher Shawn Achor, psychologist Michelle Gielan, and Arianna Huffington suggested it was essential. In their research, the team randomly assigned 110 participants to two groups. One group watched three minutes of negative news before 10 a.m. Meanwhile, the second group watched three minutes of solution-focused news that communicated stories of inspiring human resilience, such as a seventy-year-old man who received his GED after failing dozens of times. Their results were staggering, finding that participants who were shown just three minutes of negative news were 27 percent more likely to report their emotional state as "unhappy" six to eight hours later compared with the second group. The team concluded that "just a few minutes spent consuming negative news in the morning can affect the entire emotional trajectory of your day."[6]

After reading the research, I couldn't ignore the importance of how we start each day. And I'll admit, part of me fell in love with the idea of crafting the Pinterest-perfect morning where I would watch the sunrise in my coordinating yoga gear while sipping a delicious green juice. However, given my current reality was hitting snooze and retreating into the comfort of my duvet, this seemed like a stretch. So, I began to research simple, easy to implement morning routines that could cultivate positive emotions and lay the foundation for flow. A few weeks into my research, I discovered the art of gratitude.

THE ART OF GRATITUDE

Over the centuries, philosophers, researchers, religious leaders, spiritual gurus, and individuals have praised the benefits of expressing what we're grateful for. According to Cicero, "Gratitude is not only the greatest of virtues, but the parent of all the others." But what exactly does "gratitude" mean? And are there any proven benefits of this practice?

While definitions of gratitude vary widely, for me, gratitude is best defined as the deep appreciation for everyday life. This mood-enhancing habit isn't about seeing the world through "rose-tinted glasses" or a strategy for self-deception; rather, the practice of gratitude encourages you to become consciously abundant. There are, of course, numerous ways to practice gratitude. However, I chose the practice of journaling for Morning Grateful Flow because it's convenient, simple, and has proven benefits.

Gratitude journaling involves writing down three things you are grateful for every day. Regardless of whether you're on vacation, a business trip, or in the middle of a busy week where you don't have much time to invest in yourself, all you need is a pen, paper, and your thoughts. And although gratitude is not a new concept, the recent advances in scientific research on the impact of gratitude are. Let's begin with understanding the effect gratitude has on your brain.

GRATITUDE AND YOUR BRAIN

The practice of gratitude encourages you to notice the little things, recall happy memories, and appreciate the beauty of now. As you engage in this act, your brain releases powerful feel-good chemicals. Practicing Morning Grateful Flow every day is like taking a neurological super smoothie that helps boosts your happiness for the day, incorporating the following ingredients:

A Dollop of Dopamine: The practice of gratitude has been linked to increased dopamine levels in your brain.[7] Dopamine gives you that feel-good factor and increases your motivation levels. Better yet, the feel-good factor encourages you to repeat an activity, which means practicing Morning Grateful Flow doesn't require a huge amount of additional effort.

A Cup of Confirmation Bias: Confirmation bias refers to a phenomenon studied by neuroscientists and psychologists who have found that our brains favor what we already believe. This means that the more you notice things to be grateful for, the more your brain will actively seek out these things. As the neuroscientist Alex Korb explains in *Psychology Today*, "Your brain loves to fall for the confirmation bias, that is it looks for things that prove what it already believes to be true. . . . So once you start seeing things to be grateful for, your brain starts looking for more things to be grateful for."[8]

A Heap of Hypothalamus Activity: Gratitude has been shown to stimulate activity in the hypothalamus—a small but very important part of the brain.[9] The hypothalamus keeps your entire bodily system in check, balances hormones, and plays a key role in stress regulation and sleep.

And the benefits don't end there. It's not only what happens inside your brain that makes gratitude powerful, but it's also how these inward changes manifest outwardly in your everyday life that is truly amazing.

Gratitude is associated with improved physical health.
A study found that undergraduate health psychology students who were asked to journal five things weekly they were grateful for for ten weeks exercised significantly more and reported fewer physical complaints compared to students who were asked to journal five annoyances.[10]
A comprehensive white paper by The Greater Good Science Center at UC Berkeley on the science of gratitude cited other studies that linked gratitude to including improved sleep, reduced biomarkers for inflammation in heart failure patients, and less burnout.[11]

Studies have found that gratitude improves romantic relationships. Psychologist Sarah Algoe and her colleagues found that grateful couples reported greater levels of satisfaction and connection. Their study concluded that everyday gratitude might act as a "booster shot" for romantic relationships.[12]

Gratitude is linked to achievements at work. Studies have linked gratitude with increased levels of job satisfaction[13] and higher levels of performance at work.[14]

THE FEEL-GOOD FACTOR
AND FLOW

When we feel good, we are able to focus with greater ease because our energy is not wasted on worry, fear, or doubt. This ability to focus our attention in the present is vital for flow, and a positive emotional state plays a valuable role in this. As Mihaly Csikszentmihalyi explains in his book *Finding Flow: The Psychology of Engagement with Everyday Life*, being in a positive emotional state means "psychic energy can flow freely into whatever thought or task we choose to invest it in."[15] His expert views are supported by the extensive research of psychologist Alice M. Isen and her colleagues, who found that when you feel positive emotions, you display thought patterns that facilitate creative problem-solving,[16] flexibility,[17] and thoroughness.[18] Conversely, it has been proposed that when you experience negative emotions, your ability to focus decreases[19]—it's this narrowing of attention that may cause you to miss opportunities.

Morning Grateful Flow lets you take responsibility for your morning mood, helping you cultivate positive emotions at the start of each day and lay the foundation to find your flow.

HOW TO PRACTICE MORNING GRATEFUL FLOW

The practice of Morning Grateful Flow helps cultivate and sustain a positive emotional state, and being in this state helps create the optimal conditions for finding your flow. This simple, evidence-based practice just takes a few minutes to do at the start of each day. Here's how to get started:

1. First thing in the morning, before checking your phone, find a quiet space and take out a journal/notebook and a pen.

2. Taking three deep breaths to center yourself, write down three things you're grateful for in your life right now. This could be a relationship, something that happened the day before, an aspect of nature, a person in your life, etc.

3. Gratitude is an emotion, so really feel it as you write down your statements. For example, smile as you remember how grateful you are for your health and the beautiful park you go for a run in. To enhance the emotion, try visualizing the person or situation you are grateful for—really feel how you felt, see what you saw, and hear what you heard.

GRATITUDE
101

GRATITUDE IS NOT . . .

- Comparing yourself to others (e.g., I'm so grateful that my car didn't break down like Eve's car did.).

- Wishful thinking (e.g., I'll be grateful when I own my new house or go on an extravagant vacation or start my own business).

GRATITUDE IS . . .

- A powerful celebration of all you have in this present moment.

- A practice that requires patience. Like any new practice, it takes time. Be gentle with yourself if you feel like you "aren't getting it." Stick with it, and it will come.

- Important to practice in tough times. A study identified the trait of gratitude as one of the positive coping strategies people applied in challenging times.[20]

THE RIPPLE EFFECT

Now, let's fast-forward to the present day where you won't find me endlessly scrolling on my phone in the mornings; instead, I reach for my journal. Taking my pen, a smile stretches across my face as I write about how grateful I am for my husband, Chris, and his love, support, and friendship. I write about how grateful I am for last night's dinner with friends where I laughed so hard, I cried. And I recall with gratitude a walk where I drank my favorite coffee and felt the winter sun warm my skin as it glistened through the trees.

I've found that no matter how frantic my week is, my Morning Grateful Flow practice grounds me. This ritual fills me with feelings of inner peace, joy, and connection to the world around me. It has opened my eyes to the beauty in the small moments that surround us each day, making me truly grateful for life.

Morning Grateful Flow is your morning reminder that everything you need is already here. It's a welcomed pause that enables you to absorb life for all that it is. And as you gently descend into a new day with positive energy, the ripple effect of how to find your flow begins.

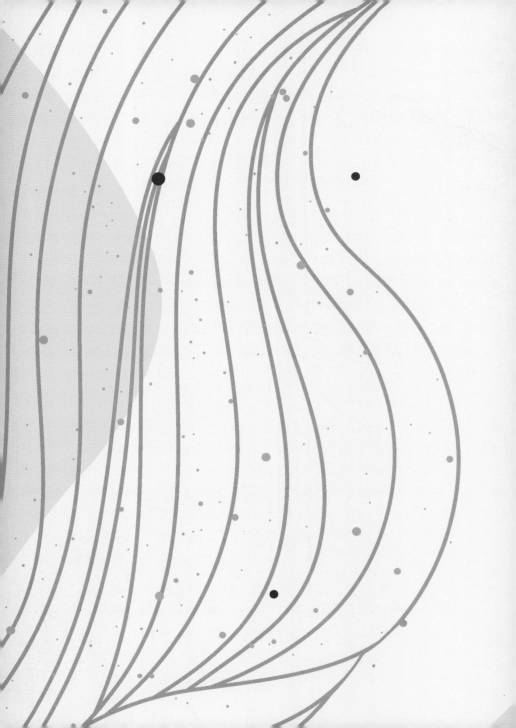

FORWARD FOCUS:
LIVE WITH INTENTION

As the ripples of gratitude rise
To greet the energy of the day
Resistance dissolves and
Clarity casts over
Possibilities
Priorities
And
Curiosity
Of what could be
As you slide into the
current of your flow with

FORWARD FOCUS

CAUGHT IN THE BUSY TRAP

As I sip my second cup of coffee, I tell my friend Cathy, "I really need this to get me through today. I'm so busy right now."

And it's the truth. It's a few months until my thirty-fouth birthday and my feelings of being overwhelmed and lack of control are rising.

Sitting at our table in an overpriced, uber-trendy coffee shop, I watch as Cathy's mouth moves up and down, telling me about her new job. And although I catch fragments of what she is saying, most of her words wash over me. My smiling facade conceals the invisible war raging in my head as my never-ending priorities jostle and vie for power. This mental tug-of-war pushes and pulls my focus in different directions, causing me to feel overwhelmed and out of balance. I take another swig of coffee in the desperate hope that it will perk me up.

During this time in my life, it felt like everything was a priority that demanded my attention. I needed to slow down, re-evaluate, and understand where to best channel my energy. But truthfully, I was scared to stop, because if I did, I'd have to face the uncomfortable question that was in the back of my mind: Am I doing what matters or am I wasting my time?

New York Times journalist Tim Kreider calls this modern phenomenon "the busy trap,"[21] and I was caught up in it. He says that people are "busy because of their own ambition or drive or anxiety because they're addicted to busyness and dread what they might have to face in its absence."[22] In her book Daring Greatly, researcher and author Brené Brown shares a similar view that we "are a culture of people who've bought into the idea that if we stay busy enough, the truth of our lives won't catch up with us."[23]

As I sat sipping coffee, little did I know that in a matter of weeks, the truth of my life would catch up with me and knock me off my feet with one simple question.

THE QUESTION THAT CHANGED EVERYTHING

I took my seat in a crowded theater. It was a beautiful spring evening, and I had decided to try and ease feeling over-whelmed with some inspiration at a motivational seminar. As I sat in the crowd feeling uplifted and inspired, the presenter floored me by asking one question that completely changed my perspective: "Can you name three activities you like to do in your leisure time? This is about what *you* do for no other reason than that these activities make you happy and give you a sense of purpose."

My mind was completely blank, and I couldn't think of an answer. I'd been so busy that I'd somehow disconnected from what I wanted. I felt confused. What did I like? What gave me purpose?

I watched as those around me frantically wrote in their notepads. Feeling ashamed and embarrassed by my empty page, I scribbled the only three things I could think of: swimming, walking, and reading (the same three imaginary hobbies I'd written on my resume over ten years ago).

I returned home, haunted by that question and my inability to answer it. I wanted to pass it off as a silly question or justify my inability to answer it with a roll of my eyes and sarcastic reply of "I wish I could do the things I loved—if I only had the time." Instead of making excuses, I stood in the light of my truth and admitted that while I was "so busy" doing everything, I wasn't accomplishing anything of real importance.

GIVING YOURSELF THE GIFT OF TIME

When life gets busy, you can find yourself being influenced by other people's priorities, hurried along by their timeline of success, or floundering under the self-inflicted pressure to have the "instant success" that is fed to you through social media every day. It's easy to get caught up in the resistance of these pressures. As editor of the *Johns Hopkins Health Review*, Elizabeth Evitts Dickinson, observes, "There's a global epidemic of overscheduling and it's ruining our health."[24] In my own life, I had become an unnecessary martyr, refusing to give myself permission to slow down and let life in. I was locked away in a self-created purgatory, torturing myself daily with the thought that I wasn't good enough.

But taking a step back from the complexities of modern life revealed a simple truth: understanding and making time for your goals and priorities determine the quality and meaning of your life. Indeed, psychologists claim that "without goals, life would lack structure and purpose"[25] and have found that people with goals report higher levels of life satisfaction and happiness.[26]

Curious about how goals and flow are related, I turned to Mihaly Csikszentmihalyi's research on flow for answers once again. Were there any clues in his research that would consistently set me free from the busy trap?

FOCUS AND FLOW

Csikszentmihalyi found that people who experience flow have clear goals and an optimal level of challenge (two of the three core conditions to foster flow). Applying this to my everyday life, I wondered if I could find flow in setting priorities (clear goals) and completing them to the best of my current ability (optimal level of challenge).

It sounded relatively straightforward, but what about the priorities in life that were must-dos, such as paying bills, cooking, shopping, and cleaning? Was there an opportunity to find flow in these activities? With Csikszentmihalyi concluding that "almost any activity can produce flow provided the relevant elements are present, it is possible to improve the quality of life by making sure that . . . [the] conditions of flow are as much as possible a constant part of everyday life,"[27] I felt confident that I could find a way to intentionally structure my day around conditions that fostered flow. And after a lot of experimenting, I developed Forward Focus.

FORWARD FOCUS

Forward Focus is the second part of your morning ritual to find your flow. It integrates two of the core conditions for flow—clear goals and optimal level of challenge—into everyday life.

Forward Focus will trade your busyness for intention and ensure that the time you have is well spent. Forward Focus is used to align your daily priorities with your big life goals (creating unified flow) and increase your daily activities where you feel in flow (increasing flow experiences). It can be completed in three simple steps:

1. Set three daily goals you must do (high-value priorities).
2. Set three daily goals you want to do (high-flow priorities).
3. Write down your schedule for the day to bring greater awareness of how you use your time.

To make sure you gain maximum value from this powerful practice, we will dive a little deeper into each step and explore how you can add in the optimal level of challenge to find your flow.

SETTING YOUR DAILY GOALS:
HIGH-VALUE PRIORITIES

There are things that you must do in your daily life, such as take a closer look at your finances, go food shopping, meet work deadlines, exercise, or have a difficult conversation with a friend or coworker. While these priorities aren't particularly inspiring and are sometimes uncomfortable, they are necessary to prevent future problems, such as debt, poor health, or the downfall of relationships. So, although you may not always have a choice in **what** you must do, you have a choice in **how** you do it.

> **Choice 1:** Use your precious time and energy to complain about your responsibilities. You can moan about it for most of the day, tell people how you don't want to do it, and generally make it as uncomfortable for yourself as possible. When you finally engage in the task, you can sigh (a lot), and if you really want to punish yourself, try repeating the words "When is this going to be finished"? over and over in your head. Generally, resist the present moment as much as possible and use your mental energy to wish it away.

> **Choice 2:** Approach what you must do with acceptance as you work with it, not against it. Release the tight grip of resistance and allow the present moment to flow. There is no need to force yourself to love what you're doing or label it as "good" or "bad"—it just simply is. Acceptance of the present moment reserves your precious time and energy for more of what really matters in life.

Each morning, when you set your high-value priorities, you instantly bring awareness to what you must do so that you can approach it with greater acceptance, flowing around it instead of resisting it.

What type of activities should be on your high-value priorities list? These are the priorities you must do and that add the most value to your life. This could be submitting a job application, doing your shopping, logging your expenses, scheduling a dentist appointmetnt, or making that call you have been avoiding all week.

How many high-value priorities should you set? I suggest you select three high-value priorities each day to maintain focus and prevent feeling overwhelmed. This may mean you'll have to relentlessly prioritize what's important. If you're struggling to streamline to only three, try using these questions to help you determine what's best to focus on:

- What would happen if I don't complete this high-value priority?

- Is it possible to delegate this to someone else?

- Am I completing this out of guilt or obligation? What would happen if I said no?

- Is this task necessary?

- Does this high-value priority need my attention today or can it wait?

- Can it be broken down into smaller, more manageable tasks?

- What will completing this high-value priority do for me? How does it make my life and work better?

TIP: When it comes to your high-value priorities, ask yourself what you can change or add to make them more enjoyable. How can you make these activities less of a chore?

SETTING YOUR DAILY GOALS:
HIGH-FLOW PRIORITIES

High-flow priorities are the activities that give you a sense of flow. They are typically activities that you want to do or activities where you feel in flow. They are daily goals that encourage you to become curious and find your flow in work and leisure time. And as you notice when flow happens, high-flow priorities will provide the structure to purposefully make flow happen more. In order to find your flow, it's vital that you use these priorities to become curious about life and work, experiment with your passions, notice when you feel in flow, and seek out clues that guide you to your true purpose. High-flow priorities are a daily reminder that you are in control of your experience and can structure your day to feel the rewards from doing what you love.

What type of activities should be on your high-flow priorities list? High-flow priorities are daily goals where you feel in flow and that are in alignment with your bigger life goals. They give you the joy of flow experiences, as well as the serenity and meaning that come from living in unified flow, and make the best use of your time and potential. For example, one high-flow priority may be to spend thirty minutes writing because you have always wanted to publish a book. Your second might be giving a presentation on a new product at work, because it's here that you feel "in the zone." And your third high-flow priority might be trying a new dance class, as you're curious to see if you'll feel a sense of flow. High-flow priorities also offer a space for self-care and can be as simple as going for a short walk, reading a book, taking a candlelit bubble bath, or going to the cinema. Ultimately, it's your responsibility to create the structure of your day, decide how you will take small daily steps toward your bigger goals, and choose the content of your experience of life.

TIP: Activities that lend their structure to the conditions of flow, such as games, sports, and the arts, are great ways to add and experience flow in your life. Think about how you could integrate these things by hosting a game night, taking a climbing lesson, or a trying your hand at painting.

How many high-flow priorities should you set? As with high-value priorities, I suggest you set three high-flow priorities to maintain focus. However, you might get stuck thinking about what you *don't* want to do, making it difficult to turn your attention toward what you *do* want to do. If you're struggling to think of things you want to do or are having trouble identifying when you are in flow, try answering these questions to get started:

- What life experiences do you want to have? What small steps can you take today that will move you toward the life you want to live?

- What type of activities make you happy? Are there games you enjoy or gym classes you love?

- What leisure activities give you meaning, purpose, and joy?

- What type of tasks do you become completely absorbed in at work?

- What activities make you lose your sense of time and self?

- When do you feel in flow (total engagement) at work? How could you add more of this into your workday to increase your level of job satisfaction?

- What did you enjoy doing as a child?

- What do you do because you love it (not for money or any form of reward)?

- What could you do to show yourself some self-love today?

It's vital to develop a curiosity about what makes you happy. Take the time to experiment and notice when you feel in alignment, and you'll find the answers and your own flow.

TIP: If you're struggling with what you want to do or where you find flow, try challenging yourself to write a list of one hundred things you enjoy. You'll be surprised at what you write and the themes you spot.

SETTING YOUR SCHEDULE

The act of setting a schedule will determine when and where you'll complete your priorities. Adhering to a schedule moves you from a daily goal to a daily action, while bringing conscious awareness to how and where you use your precious gift of time. Research tells us that the simple act of just thinking about time motivates us to engage in behaviors associated with greater happiness levels, such as spending more time with friends and family.[28]

What if your schedule doesn't go as planned? A big part of being in flow is learning to surrender and let go when things happen that are outside your control. If things aren't unfolding as you planned, observe them as they are, accept them, and release your resistance of wanting the present moment to be something that it's not. And if your schedule

FINDING YOUR OPTIMAL LEVEL OF CHALLENGE

"Enjoyment appears at the boundary between boredom and anxiety, when challenges are just balanced with the person's capacity to act."

—Mihaly Csikszentmihalyi, *Flow*

Finding the right level of challenge for flow involves fine-tuning the balance between your skills and the level of challenge. When you find your optimal level of challenge—not too difficult that you feel anxious and not too easy that you feel bored—flow occurs. It's here that your awareness merges with your action, as you become lost in the total involvement of your task. If an activity feels too boring or mundane, increase the level of challenge. For example, set a time challenge or try to beat your previous performance. If your routine is causing you to feel bored, think of ways to challenge yourself in order to get back into flow. Similarly, if an activity is making you feel anxious,try decreasing the level of challenge. For example, if you want to start a business but it feels too overwhelming, start with an online course or go to an event. Or if you want to increase your fitness but a gym class feels too daunting, try a home workout or go for a walk.

doesn't go as planned because of your own limiting beliefs or unwanted habits, get curious and explore how you can learn from this experience.

SCHEDULING FOR SUCCESS

Setting your schedule can foster flow and keep your brain healthy and happy. Here are a few points to consider when setting and completing your daily schedule:

Do one thing at a time. There is a modern misconception that it's better to multitask in order to get more done; however, this is not your brain's preferred way of working. Neuroscience and psychology tell us that multitasking can make you up to 40 percent less productive.[29] Furthermore, switching from one task to another makes you feel tired more quickly, as it depletes glucose levels, an essential fuel for effective brain function.[30] So, when setting your schedule, make a "one-task-at-a-time" rule.

Build in transition time between tasks. Creating space in your schedule in between tasks or activities can help you mindfully transition from one task to the next.

Minimize interruptions. Beware of the distraction thieves, as their seemingly harmless "Do you have a minute?" interruptions cost valuable time. In fact, Professor Gloria Mark found it took an average of twenty-three minutes and fifteen seconds to resume a task after being interrupted.[31] When setting your schedule, consider how you can minimize interruptions to enhance focus and flow. Perhaps you can wear headphones at work, find a quiet space to ground yourself, or simply ask others to refrain from interrupting you unless it's urgent.

Limit screen time. Without question, smartphones, tablets, and electronic devices are the top modern-day distractions. As you scroll through social media, it's easy to get lost in a never-ending vacuum of articles, videos, and updates. To stay focused and on task, set your phone on airplane mode and activate the timer. The timer can add the optimal level of challenge, encouraging you to get a task done in a set amount of time.

HOW TO PRACTICE FORWARD FOCUS

Practice Forward Focus immediately after Morning Grateful Flow. Here's how to do it:

1. Set three daily goals you must do (high-value priorities). They can be simple statements, like "register for the online training I want to complete" or "send the holiday request form to my manager."

2. Set three daily goals you want to do (high-flow priorities). Again, these can be simple statements, like "go for a walk in the park on my lunch break" or "attend a local improv class."

3. Write out your schedule for the day. It helps to write out each hour of the day, indicating the times when you will complete your high-value and high-flow priorities. You may be surprised by how much awareness this brings to how you use your time.

4. Review and rework your schedule, especially if you find you've overscheduled your day.

A LIFE OF MEANING

Forward Focus changed my life. It enabled me to develop the daily habit of ordering my priorities, aligning with my purpose, and enjoying the journey. But beyond those things, it helped me develop healthy boundaries, say no with grace, discover passions, accept rather than resist the present moment, and develop a deep curiosity about life. This practice has slowed down life and brought a sense of inner control, as it allows me to meaningfully focus on what matters most. After all, there is no better way to design your future than to focus on how you are using your time and potential in the present.

Forward Focus will help you flow throughout the day as you set clear goals that challenge you—you learn to embrace all that you are and all that you are becoming. Continuing the ripple effect, Forward Focus ensures that the far-reaching effects of your everyday actions create the fulfilling, meaningful life you seek.

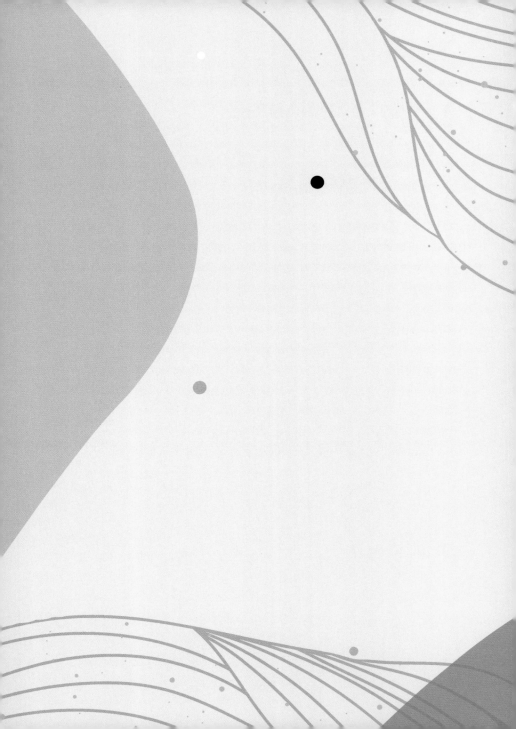

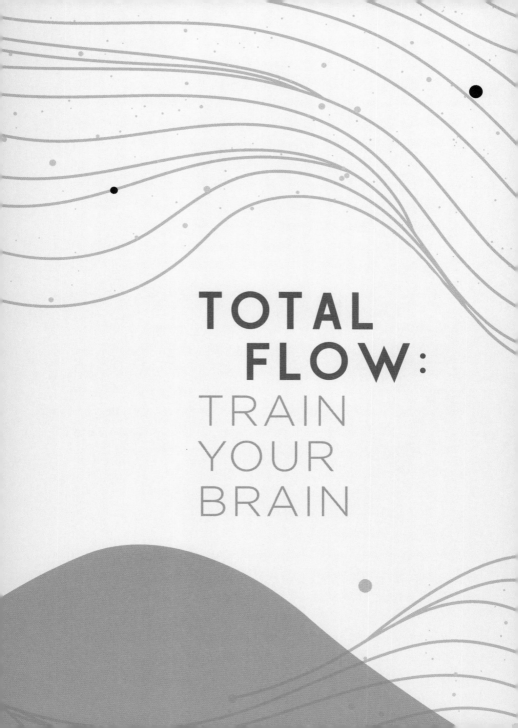

TOTAL FLOW:
TRAIN YOUR BRAIN

Time flows
The day unravels
And those who flow
Are both
accepting and prepared
For the challenges that will arise
And the distractions
that will transpire
They know that left unguarded
The current of life can sweep
them off course
So they remain rooted
In their own story
and unique current with

TOTAL FLOW

IT TAKES MORE THAN GOOD INTENTIONS

I peer up from my laptop and watch as my colleagues file into my office, as they enthusiastically sing "Happy Birthday." I force a smile.

I had pictured my thirty-fourth birthday to be so different. I'd imagined myself fitter and healthier by this age. I had wanted to write a book, travel, and start prioritizing my dreams. And yet, I was another year older with the same good intentions and familiar weight of disappointment in my life choices. Frustrated, angst-ridden, and unconvinced by my own inner chatter that this year will be different, I was depleted by my desire to be more. I wondered, *Perhaps it would be easier if I simply gave up.* How could I feel happy and full in the present and take meaningful action toward the goals I desired in the future?

I don't think my story is an unfamiliar one, and I believe there are a growing number of people who silently struggle under the often-invisible weight of an unfulfilled life. But why is it so easy to get distracted and pulled away from your goals? Why does it feel so hard to create a meaningful life you want and deserve?

YOUR ATTENTION IS UNDER ATTACK

Your attention is precious, selective, and limited. And in the current technological age, human attention and focus are in demand more than ever before. From the moment you open your eyes, an army of "attention thieves" are poised and ready to attack. They lurk in your missed notifications, app messages, news threads, email inbox, social media feeds, and those hilarious dog videos.

But don't be fooled, for this is a coordinated attack. These "attention thieves" have been strategically placed to deliberately divert your attention, because the more time you spend clicking and scrolling, the more online ads you're exposed to and the more data you share. As the adage goes, "There's no such thing as a free lunch," and in today's modern economy, attention is currency.

Tristan Harris, a former Google employee, shares his insight into the growing number of distraction tactics created by this "attention economy"[32] in his TED Talk "How a Handful of Tech Companies Control Billions of Minds Every Day." As a design ethicist, Tristan's job was to study how to influence people's thoughts. He warns, "What we don't talk about is how the handful of people working at a handful of technology companies . . . will steer what a billion people are thinking today. Because when you pull out your phone and they design how this works or what's on the feed, it's scheduling little blocks of time in our minds. If you see a notification, it schedules you to have thoughts that maybe you didn't intend to have."[33]

And their strategies are working. According to the *New York Times*, more than three-quarter of all Americans (253 million people) spent 1,460 hours on their smartphones and other mobile devices in 2018. Those hours total nine-ty-one waking days or a collective 370 billion waking hours lost to screen time.[34]

But before you retreat into the wilderness and go off the grid, the good news is you can train your attention to manage distractions, technological or otherwise. In the same way the first step to developing better nutritional health is an awareness of how your body processes food, the first step to better attentional health is understanding how your mind processes information.

YOUR ATTENTION:
THE GATEKEEPER TO YOUR MEANINGFUL LIFE

Your attention is the powerful gatekeeper to your conscious-ness. Tasked with differentiating what information is most relevant or irrelevant, it plays a vital role in creating your experience of life. Like a doorman working at an exclusive nightclub, your attention dutifully ushers the most useful information into your "consciousness party" every 250 milliseconds.[35] As each informational guest arrives, you interact with them, gaining valuable feedback that shapes the content and meaning of your life. And when your attention functions optimally, it can throw the perfect party. It filters in "guests" that spark creative ideas, deep connection, and meaning. However, the increasing demand on your attention's limited resources means it's working under challenging conditions.

In a fascinating study, Martin Hilbert and Priscila López quantified the increase in the amount of information sloshing about in our environment between 1986 and 2007. Their jaw-dropping statistics show the scale of the challenge your attention is facing:

- People shared 65 exabytes of information in 2007 via telecommunications, which is comparable to every person in the world sending out the contents of 6 newspapers every day.

- In 2007, we globally broadcast almost 2 zettabytes of information, which is the equivalent of every person in the world reading 174 newspapers each day.

- And telecommunications have grown 28 percent annually since 1986.[36]

Your attention—an overwhelmed and distracted gatekeeper—stands between this barrage of information and your consciousness. When pushed to its limit, your attention will wane like a stressed employee drowning in a sea of paperwork. Its limited nature and finite resource mean that the demands to "hustle harder" or "push through" will only have an adverse effect. As your attention struggles to differentiate between what's relevant and irrelevant, unwanted "guests" will inevitably nudge their way into your conscious awareness. Social media comparison will make you feel inadequate, distractions will take you off schedule, and emails will signal the urgency of other people's priorities. In the same way junk food consumes your calorie budget, "junk information" consumes your capacity to pay attention.

In his book *Optimal Experience: Psychological Studies of Flow in Consciousness*, Mihaly Csikszentmihalyi estimates that your brain can process 126 bits of information per second. While this might sound like a lot, a third of this capacity is used just by listening to a conversation. He explains, "In a lifetime of seventy years, assuming a waking day of sixteen hours, this amounts to 185 billion bits of information. This number defines the limit of individual experience. Out of it must come every perception, thought, feeling, memory, or action that a person will ever have. It seems like a large number, but in actuality most people find it tragically insufficient."[37]

To craft a life of meaning, you need to have a greater awareness of how you're spending your attention budget. Just like with nutritional health, where you are what you eat, with attentional health, you become what you pay attention to. If you could achieve mastery over one skill that would radically shape the quality and content of your experience, it's your attention. It's the ability to move and apply your attention at will that shapes and connects your experience of your outer and inner worlds.

The power of attention enables a writer to craft masterpieces, an inventor to invent life-changing creations, and a musician to construct melodies that speak to the soul. It allows you to shift from the trauma of the past to the possibilities of the future. In short, whatever you choose to shine your spotlight of attention on becomes part of your experience and will shape your unique perception of reality. As the psychologist William James observed, "Experience is what I agree to attend to. Only those items which I notice shape my mind."[38]

You are surrounded by feedback. It comes in the forms of how you feel, what you hear, and what you see. Feedback is a powerful tool that can help you recognize what's important to pay attention to and what's not. Feedback cues are the micro-moments that signal whether you're on the right course or need to adjust your actions. For example, if you are in a job interview, your brain will receive positive feedback when the interviewer smiles and nods at your answers—a feedback cue that you are on track— or negative feedback if the interviewer looks confused or bored—a feedback cue that you should read just your actions.

As Ian Fiebelkorn, an associate research scholar at the Princeton Neuroscience Institute, explains, "Every 250 milliseconds, you have an opportunity to switch attention. You won't necessarily shift your focus to a new subject but your brain has a chance to re-examine your priorities and decide if it wants to."[39] The better you are at detecting these micro-moments of feedback, the greater control you will have to shift your attention and shape the content of your life experience.

TOTAL FLOW: THE STORY YOU WANT YOUR LIFE TO TELL

Elite athletes are masters of attention, and the techniques they use can provide valuable insight into how you can better direct and control your attention in everyday life. There is a growing recognition that while sports are physical, the game is won in the mind. And it's an athlete's ability to train their selective attention—focusing on important feedback cues and drowning out distractions—that's integral to a successful performance.[40] Sports psychologists use a process called "imagery scripting" to help athletes quickly recognize relevant feedback cues.

Imagery scripting is designed to prime an athlete's attention before an event by training their attention to focus on what's important and ignore what is irrelevant. Athletes usually work with a coach to prepare detailed written scripts that tell athletes what feedback to look for, such as the tightening of their core as they make a turn, a focus point as they approach a starting line, or the physical feeling of calm under pressure. These vivid descriptions enable athletes to mentally train their attention and become more present in the moment.

Going beyond visualization, imagery scripting intentionally embraces all the senses. Each individualized script depicts, in detail, the athlete's ideal performance. As aerial skier and Olympian Emily Cook explains in a *New York Times* interview,

"You have to smell it. You have to hear it. You have to feel it, everything."[41] Sports psychologist Nicole Detling adds, "The more an athlete can image the entire package, the better it's going to be," and she continues to say that when you script, "it's absolutely crucial that you don't fail."[42]

Imagery scripting guides an athlete's attention toward where they want it to flow, and it serves to replace negative talk, like "I won't fall over on the third jump" with "I will hurdle the third jump." When this negativity is replaced with positively framed imagery scripting, the athlete is more likely to perform at their optimal level.

More than just an anecdotal ritual, these multisensory written scripts are a highly effective guidance system proven to eliminate distractions, increase focus, and enhance flow.[43] And this technique isn't restricted to elite athletes such as the Olympian swimmer Michael Phelps. Sports psychologists claim that "all individuals, regardless of age, gender, or skill level, are capable of using imagery as a means to enhance cognitive, behavioral, and effective outcomes."[44]

Total Flow adapts imagery scripting to suit your everyday life as you describe what you will see, hear, and feel throughout your ideal day. You will learn to identify the feedback cues that communicate what's important to pay attention to. This helps drown out distraction, find your flow, and focus on what's most important. It's the morning practice that helps ensure you make the most out of your attentional budget.

HOW TO PRACTICE TOTAL FLOW

Practice Total Flow immediately after Forward Focus to engage your senses and essentially script what you'll see, hear, and feel as your ideal day working toward your priorities unfolds. By creating these clear feedback cues, you will develop a guidance system that helps your attention focus on what's useful. You don't need to script your entire day, just the parts that are most important to you. Here's how you do it:

1. In a journal or notebook, write your imagery script of your ideal day, working toward your high-value and high-flow priorities. What do you want your day to look like? How do you want to feel? What will you see, hear, and feel that will give your attention evidence that you are positively progressing to achieving your high-value and high-flow priorities?

2. Remember, energy goes where attention flows, so focus on what you want and avoid negatives (e.g., "I feel strong, calm, and confident as I head into my new dance class," as opposed to "I don't feel anxious or worried as I head into my new dance class").

3. Use positive and empowering words to describe your state (e.g., confident, motivated, strong, relaxed, centered).

4. Total Flow can be as long or as short as you want. It can cover the whole day or just parts of it. You can script all your priorities or focus on a specific priority that's significant that day. It's up to you to experiment and find what works for you.

5. After you've finished, take three deep breaths to center yourself and read through your script.

6. Close your notebook or journal and place it beside your bed. This will act as a visual reminder to complete Nighttime Reflection at the end of the day.

TIP: Total Flow is an effective tool to overcome challenges or unwanted behavior. You can do this by scripting feedback cues into your day to help embed new habits. For example, if you feel that you are using social media too much, you may script, "I notice how good it feels to use my social media with intention," or if you are having problems with a friend or work colleague, you may script, "I hear myself speak calmly today. I notice how I take time to listen to their point of view and feel calm, focused, and relaxed as we work together to resolve our problem."

TOTAL FLOW: USEFUL PHRASES AND PROMPTS

In Total Flow, you script your ideal day, writing what feedback you will see, hear, and feel as the most important parts of your day unfold. Here are some useful prompts and phrases to help with your scripting.

Prompts

- What do you see yourself or other people doing that provides feedback that you are moving toward your priorities?

- What do you hear yourself or others saying that provides feedback that you are moving toward your priorities?

- How do you want to feel?

- Consider when and where you are—and if it's helpful describe the environment.

Phrases

- I notice how . . .

- I see myself . . .

- I hear others say to me . . .

- I hear myself say . . .

- I notice the feelings of . . . when I . . .

- I notice how good it feels when I . . .

ABSORBED IN THE TOTAL FLOW OF LIFE

Feedback is one of the core conditions for flow, as identified by Mihaly Csikszentmihalyi, and it plays a vital role in communicating with your attention. But recognizing important feedback cues in our information-overloaded world is a challenge. Total Flow, the final part of your morning routine, will help you recognize feedback, control your attention, and find your flow. The process of Total Flow can help you learn how to train and control your selective attention in a similar way to athletes. Just as a chess player knows their next move, a rock climber knows where to place their foot, and a dancer knows their next turn, you, too, will know exactly where to next place your attention. This increased alignment between your intention and your attention opens the door to your own intuition. The more you become in tune with your own internal compass, the more confident you will become in charting your own course.

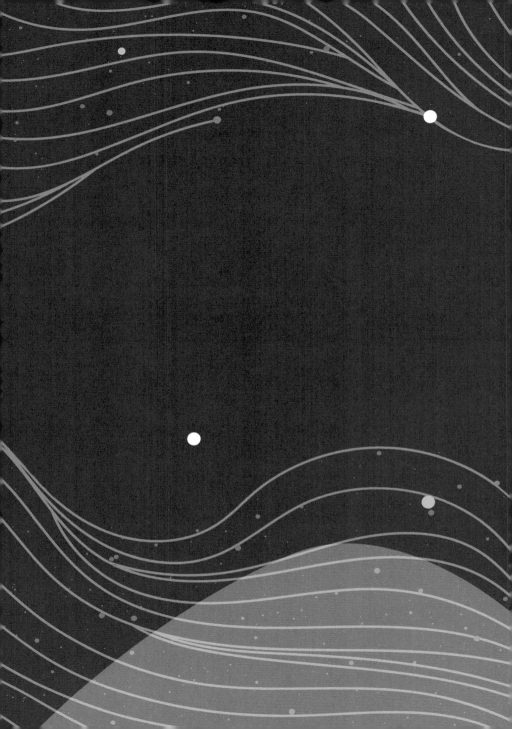

NIGHTTIME REFLECTION:
BECOME AWARE, GROW & FLOW

Drop by drop
The stories we weave
Trickle in
To form the body of our
experience of life
The stories of joy and
suffering
Created by us
Absorb into the fabric
of our being
Like water seeping into sand
Consciously shape your
experience
And direct your flow with

NIGHTTIME
REFLECTION

THE SEARCH
FOR MORE

Shortly after my thirty-fourth birthday, my husband and I revaluated our life together and made the decision to take the risk to live our dreams of working and traveling. My inner world had become so out of control that this dramatic change was the only way I could hit the reset button. After selling our house and belongings and quitting our jobs, I'm finally here on a beautiful beach in Malaysia. Although it seems my old hardwired thoughts and beliefs have journeyed with me.

As I walk on the beach, carrying my sandals in my hand,
I find myself worrying about the future, dwelling on the
past, and longing for success so that I can prove
to everyone that this risky decision wasn't a mistake.
Looking out toward the horizon, the words "no matter
where you go, there you are" circle around my head.

I release a long sigh, but this time, rather than pushing my thoughts down, I take a seat on the cold sand and reflect. I think about how this journey of small steps led me to this dramatic point. I consider how powerful it would have been to spot my unhelpful patterns of behavior and beliefs sooner. I reflect on how much happier I would have been if I'd taken the time to celebrate my small wins. And I think about how learning to embrace my uncomfortable thoughts and feelings would have fueled my growth, as opposed to feeling overwhelmed. While staring at the liquid red sunset, I know I've made the right decision to take a risk and live out my dream. But I also know that daily reflection is the key to developing a relationship with my intuition, staying on track with my purpose, and celebrating the beauty of small things so I can enjoy life's effortless flow.

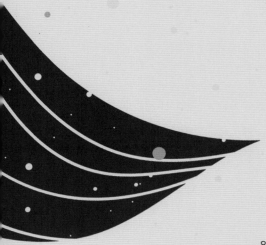

KNOW THYSELF:
THE POWER OF REFLECTION
AND SELF-AWARENESS

As far back as 2,500 years ago, the Greek philosopher Socrates said, "The unexamined life is not worth living," and his words remain prophetically relevant in our modern world. Reflection on life is an intrinsic part of our human development. Reflection is the mother of ideas, books, thoughts, music, inventions, revelations, and refinement. You have the beautiful, innate ability to be alone with your thoughts, reflect, and sculpt your internal world. Think of yourself as a "meaning maker," who can transform tragedy into purpose through the power of reflection.

Every reflection is a story that shapes each chapter of your life and molds your experience of the world around you. Although reflection is essential for personal growth, research shows that it can be an uncomfortable and somewhat unfamiliar practice for many people. Over a series of eleven studies involving more than seven hundred people, researchers found that participants typically didn't enjoy being in a room alone for six to fifteen minutes with nothing to do other than to think. The researchers found that participants would rather engage in mundane external activities or, even more surprising, numerous participants preferred to give themselves electric shocks.[45] As a result, the fear of being alone with our own thoughts has made self-awareness a rare human quality. In fact, in a recent large-scale scientific study, a team of researchers found that self-awareness was a trait present in as little as 10 to 15 percent of the five thousand people who took part.[46]

But there is value in learning to reflect and develop a strong sense of self-awareness. Science has shown that self-awareness can reap a wide range of benefits, including job-related well-being[47] and an increased likelihood of getting a promotion,[48] along with higher levels of self-esteem and self-control.[49]

Over the course of this chapter, you'll discover how to practice Nighttime Reflection for flow. You'll learn how to honestly reflect upon your life in a nonjudgmental way, gradually releasing the ideals of perfection. You'll see how to better understand your authentic self and use this knowledge to release resistance and invite change into core areas of your life. It's through reflection that you will have the courage to see, feel, and understand who you truly are and that even though life will never be perfect, you will always be enough.

THE IMPORTANCE OF A NIGHTTIME RITUAL

It may seem a little counterintuitive to practice reflection just before bed, as you may wonder if it will impact your sleep or cause worries to stir up right before bed. You may think that it's simply easier to just forget about the day and go to sleep. But research shows that writing down your problems or making to-do lists before bed is associated with a better night's sleep.[50] These findings suggest that the act of writing before bed can help unload and clear out cognitive clutter. In an interview with *Psychology Today*, psychologist Michael Scullin says, "There's something about the act of writing—physically writing something on paper. . . . The outcome seems to be that you decrease cognitive arousal and that you decrease rumination and worry."[51]

That said, it is important that you find the sweet spot on your reflection scale. If you are too quick to turn away from your problems, this can inhibit your ability to grow; conversely, if you dive in too deep, you may find yourself drowning in your worries. The sweet spot is somewhere in the middle, and it's key to find a balance in order to cultivate your ability to gently lean into your strengths and weaknesses to develop an objective curiosity about what this life lesson can teach you.

BECOMING COMFORTABLE WITH YOUR OWN THOUGHTS

In 1645, the French philosopher and mathematician Blaise Pascal wrote, "All of humanity's problems stem from man's inability to sit quietly in a room alone." And as the study at the start of this chapter reveals, there is scientific evidence to support his view that many people don't feel comfortable being alone with their own thoughts. So, how can you become more comfortable being alone with your thoughts and embracing the power of reflection? Science supports two simple tactics that can be applied through the journal process of Nighttime Reflection.

Say your name to practice self-distancing. One way to reflect on your life—and not ruminate on your problems—is to take the stance of an objective observer of your life, distancing yourself from the ego and becoming more aligned with your authentic self. Research shows that practicing self-distancing as part of self-reflection helps you think more objectively about any irrational thoughts you may have.[52] Furthermore, studies show that the "fly-on-the-wall" perspective prevents rumination and cultivates greater self-awareness.[53] The ability to distance yourself is practiced through simple changes in your language, such as shifting from the use of "I" or "my" to using your first name during self-talk to boost self-awareness.

Here's an example of how to apply this practice: Jessica was the only single person among her old school friends. The group met for dinner once a month, and Jessica adored her friends and the connection they had. Even though she was happy being single and enjoyed her active social life, she always felt different when she was with her friends, who would often talk about married life and their kids. As a result, Jessica often felt like she had nothing to contribute to the conversation and would leave feeling deflated and insecure. She'd later ruminate over the details of the evening out with her friends and create false realities in her mind.

Then, through practicing Nighttime Reflection, she learned to replace questions like "What are the reasons for *my* feelings?" with "What are the reasons for *Jessica's* feelings?" This simple switch creates linguistic distance from the self, enabling Jessica to observe her feelings, rather than become entangled in them.

As Dr. Ethan Kross, director of the Emotion and Self-Control Laboratory at the University of Michigan, explains in the *New York Times*, "If a friend comes to you with a problem it's easy to coach them through it, but if the problem is happening to us we have real difficulty, in part because we have all these egocentric biases making it hard to reason rationally." He continues, "The data clearly shows that you can use language to almost trick yourself into thinking your problems are happening to someone else."[54]

Replace "why" questions with "what" questions to increase self-awareness. The second tip to aid effective reflection comes from a fascinating study by Tasha Eurich and her team. They found that the most self-aware people don't ask "why," but they ask "what" instead. In fact, the word "why" appeared fewer than 150 times in their interviews, compared to the word "what," which appeared more than 1,000 times.[55] This subtle linguistic shift—from "why" to "what"—can have a big impact on the quality of reflection, self-awareness, and your life.

When you ask yourself "why," you instruct your brain to search for answers and to find meaning. The absence of real answers can often lead to incorrect assumptions or the fabrication of reality. If, for example, Jessica, who was feeling left out during a dinner with friends, asked herself "why" one of her friends said something, she might be inclined to create stories and false realities that would only enhance her insecurity. But if Jessica were to ask, "What are the steps *Jessica* needs to take in order to feel more secure about being single when she's out with her married friends?" this question puts her in the role of an objective observer. From this vantage point, Jessica can see herself more clearly and objectively assess and learn how to control her own reality.

THE POWER OF
SMALL STEPS

In our "quick-win" culture of instant gratification, it's easy to place more value on the destination rather than the journey. You want to get that promotion, find your purpose, meet your soul mate, get a new car, buy a house, have the perfect body—and you want it all now. Sound familiar?

But as people rush from one task to the next and are simply "getting through" the week, they dishonor the present moment and become blind to the power of taking small steps toward progress. With your eye on the prize (or destination), you focus more on what you lack, wish time away, and create resistance in your life. This resistance takes you further from your individuality and natural flow. But the practice of reflection enables you to illuminate the entire journey—honoring the present moment and letting you see the preparation you're already doing to reach your desired destination.

It's through the journal practice of Nighttime Reflection that you can celebrate small wins and recognize that the destination is an ever-moving point. You'll find that it's the ability to enjoy the current that connects each destination that gives life meaning and joy. By celebrating the strength of your small steps, you give yourself permission to enjoy the journey.

RECOGNIZE YOUR FLOW

Everyone has their own individual flow, and what elicits flow for one person may not work for another. The practice of Nighttime Reflection will help you recognize when you feel in flow so that you can integrate more of it into your life. As you practice this daily reflection, pay close attention to when you feel in flow: What time of day is it? Who are you with? What are you doing? What high-value and high-flow priorities are you working toward? As you discover these markers of your own individual current and patterns, it will become easier to recognize and rejoin the natural flow of your life, especially when you feel resistance.

Reflection plays an important role in flow, as Mihaly Csikszentmihalyi observes in his book *Finding Flow*, "It's important to find out what rhythms are most congenial to you personally . . . reflection helps to identify one's preferences and experimentation with different alternatives."[56]

TIP: A great way to track your life rhythms is to create a flow list in the back of your journal that documents the activities, people, and places that make you feel in flow. Whether it's writing, swimming, volunteering, or spending time with friends or loved one, it's important to pinpoint and experiment with what works best for you.

HOW TO PRACTICE NIGHTTIME REFLECTION

Shortly before going to sleep, find a quiet space and follow these steps:

1. Take out your journal or notebook and a pen, and reflect on your day. To do this, it's helpful to reread your morning ritual, paying particular attention to the priorities you set in Forward Focus and the script you wrote in Total Flow.

2. Write down three things that could have been better. This could be something you're worried about, a conflict, or an overpacked schedule. Be honest with yourself and bring awareness to where you are now. Take time to spot recurring lessons and lean into them, asking yourself why this is showing up in your life. What is this lesson trying to teach you? What are the opportunities for personal growth? If it helps, organize your thoughts and write them down in your journal.

3. Write down three things that you enjoyed about today. Examples include giving a great presentation at work, carving out "me time" to go to the gym, reading a book, or just being more present. Also pay attention to when you felt most in your flow during the day and think about how you can weave more of these activities into your everyday life using Forward Focus.

4. Take a deep breath, center yourself, and know that you are exactly where you are meant to be.

EVERY EXPERIENCE IS VALUABLE, EVEN THE BAD ONES

After leaving my "old" life behind, I began to research and develop the journal system for flow. Nighttime Reflection became a vital part of the system that helped me build a "new" life, keeping me on course toward what mattered most while enjoying the journey to get there. As I leaned into the small moments and took note of the life lessons that continually showed up, I could see what I needed to learn from them. I was able to track trends in my life, including the times of day I felt more productive, when and where I felt happy, and what energized me. I was getting good at creating my own story—finding and growing within my own unique flow. I learned to trust the natural rhythm of my life and no longer felt the need to rush or have everything all at once. Each step on the journey was preparing me for the next, and I appreciated the fact that I was where I was meant to be.

Nighttime Reflection is a continual practice that will keep you in your flow. It's a guidance system that will prevent you from straying too far away from the individual current of your life. It's through this process that you will cultivate more flow, integrate more activities that bring joy into your everyday experiences, and uncover the beautiful truth that the ebb and flow of life's rhythms are intrinsically connected.

Life is a dynamic contrast of highs and lows, woven together with the threads of the stories you tell yourself. You are the author of the stories, and the practice of reflection gives them life. The stories you tell about lessons learned and the blessings in unanswered prayers shape your experience of life. These stories aren't created to impress or please other people, but rather as a daily reminder that no personal experienced is wasted. Your stories are most powerful when they align with your authentic self, offering a source of strength during the hard times and a reminder of all there is to be grateful for when times are good.

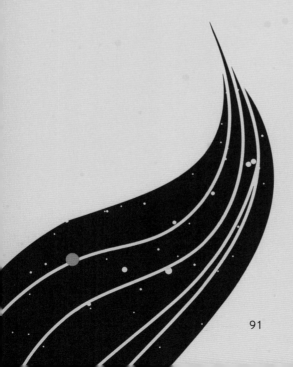

CONCLUSION

Happiness was the state I most desired in life. And up until my thirty-fourth birthday, I believed the road to success paved the way. I had diligently run along the winding road of success in search of my beloved happiness. I had pushed myself to reach many of its milestones, including education, promotions, and status. But every milestone seemed to expose another part of the road still left to run. Back then, I wanted to enjoy the process of living without abandoning my ambition and passions. I longed to feel a sense of meaning, experience joy, embrace challenge, and grow as a person. The psychology of flow showed me this was possible and developing the journal system showed me how. As I continue to combine travel and work, this daily practice has brought control, order, happiness, and flow to my life.

We all yearn to live a full, authentic, purposeful life. And I believe that people are most afraid of being "useless" as they let their talents dissolve and dreams fade. The key to living a meaningful life is to find and cultivate your unique flow.

The journal system in this book is designed to help you appreciate what you already have, act with intention toward what you want, pay attention to the everyday whispers of the universe, and lean into the lessons you're here to learn. Throughout this process, you will find your flow. And when you do, you, too, will come to understand the meaning of Lao Tzu's sentiment that "those who flow as life flows know They need no other force."

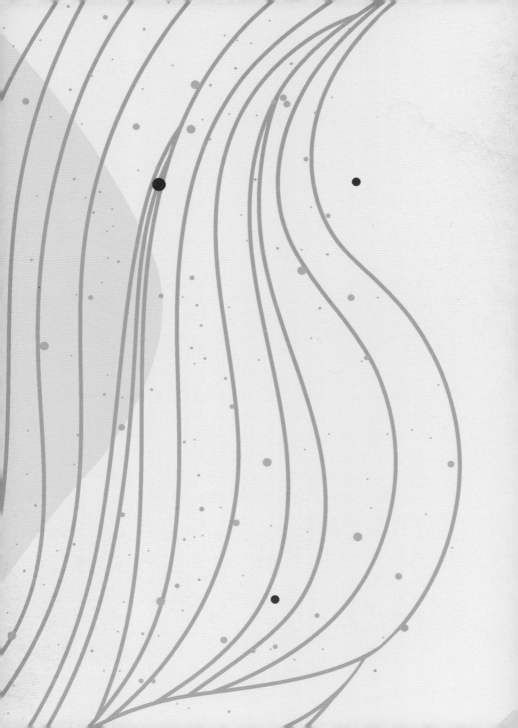

JOURNAL SUMMARY AND PAGES

FOUR-STEP JOURNAL SYSTEM SUMMARY

Here is an easy-to-access summary of the four-step journal system discussed in *Find Your Flow*. Journal pages have also been included to help get you started with your daily journaling routine. Remember, more detailed instructions can be found within each chapter.

1. Morning Grateful Flow: Wake Up Happy (page 25)
First thing in the morning, write down three things
that you are grateful for.

2. Forward Focus: Live with Intention (page 41)

- Identify three things you must do today
  (high-value priorities).

- Identify three things you want to do today
  (high-flow priorities).

- Set your schedule for the day, identifying when and
  where you will complete your high-value and high-flow
  priorities.

3. Total Flow: Train Your Brain (page 61)
Write the story of your ideal day, scripting what you will see,
hear, and feel as your day unfolds.

**4. Nighttime Reflection: Become Aware, Grow, and Flow
(page 77)**
Write down three things that could have gone better today
and three things that went well, paying particular attention
to times when you felt in flow.

I. MORNING GRATEFUL FLOW

What are you grateful for today?

1.

2.

3.

2. FORWARD FOCUS

High-Value Priorities

1.

2.

3.

High-Flow Priorities

1.

2.

3.

Daily Schedule

MORNING:

AFTERNOON:

NIGHT:

3. TOTAL FLOW

Script your ideal day:

_____

_____

_____

_____

_____

_____

_____

4. NIGHTTIME REFLECTION

Improvements   **Successes**

1. _____   1. _____

2. _____   2. _____

3. _____   3. _____

When did you feel in flow today?

_____

_____

I. MORNING GRATEFUL FLOW

What are you grateful for today?

1. _____

2. _____

3. _____

2. FORWARD FOCUS

High-Value Priorities   **High-Flow Priorities**

1. _____   1. _____

2. _____   2. _____

3. _____   3. _____

Daily Schedule

MORNING: _____

_____

AFTERNOON: _____

_____

NIGHT: _____

_____

3. TOTAL FLOW

Script your ideal day:

_____

_____

_____

_____

_____

_____

_____

4. NIGHTTIME REFLECTION

Improvements   **Successes**

1. _____   1. _____

2. _____   2. _____

3. _____   3. _____

When did you feel in flow today?

_____

_____

1. MORNING GRATEFUL FLOW

What are you grateful for today?

1. _____

2. _____

3. _____

2. FORWARD FOCUS

High-Value Priorities

1. _____

2. _____

3. _____

High-Flow Priorities

1. _____

2. _____

3. _____

Daily Schedule

MORNING: _____

_____

AFTERNOON: _____

_____

NIGHT: _____

_____

3. TOTAL FLOW

Script your ideal day:

_____

_____

_____

_____

_____

_____

_____

4. NIGHTTIME REFLECTION

Improvements	Successes
1.	1.
2.	2.
3.	3.

When did you feel in flow today?

_____

_____

I. MORNING GRATEFUL FLOW

What are you grateful for today?

1.
2.
3.

2. FORWARD FOCUS

High-Value Priorities

1.
2.
3.

High-Flow Priorities

1.
2.
3.

Daily Schedule

MORNING:

AFTERNOON:

NIGHT:

3. TOTAL FLOW

Script your ideal day:

_____

_____

_____

_____

_____

_____

_____

4. NIGHTTIME REFLECTION

Improvements   **Successes**

1. _____   1. _____

2. _____   2. _____

3. _____   3. _____

When did you feel in flow today?

_____

_____

I. MORNING GRATEFUL FLOW

What are you grateful for today?

1. _____

2. _____

3. _____

2. FORWARD FOCUS

High-Value Priorities

1. _____

2. _____

3. _____

High-Flow Priorities

1. _____

2. _____

3. _____

Daily Schedule

MORNING: _____

_____

AFTERNOON: _____

_____

NIGHT: _____

_____

3. TOTAL FLOW

Script your ideal day:

_____

_____

_____

_____

_____

_____

_____

4. NIGHTTIME REFLECTION

Improvements   **Successes**

1. _____   1. _____

2. _____   2. _____

3. _____   3. _____

When did you feel in flow today?

_____

_____

I. MORNING GRATEFUL FLOW

What are you grateful for today?

1. _____

2. _____

3. _____

2. FORWARD FOCUS

High-Value Priorities

1. _____

2. _____

3. _____

High-Flow Priorities

1. _____

2. _____

3. _____

Daily Schedule

MORNING: _____

_____

AFTERNOON: _____

_____

NIGHT: _____

_____

3. TOTAL FLOW

Script your ideal day:

_____

_____

_____

_____

_____

_____

_____

4. NIGHTTIME REFLECTION

Improvements   **Successes**

1. _____   1. _____

2. _____   2. _____

3. _____   3. _____

When did you feel in flow today?

_____

_____

1. MORNING GRATEFUL FLOW

What are you grateful for today?

1. _____

2. _____

3. _____

2. FORWARD FOCUS

High-Value Priorities   **High-Flow Priorities**

1. _____   1. _____

2. _____   2. _____

3. _____   3. _____

Daily Schedule

MORNING: _____

_____

AFTERNOON: _____

_____

NIGHT: _____

3. TOTAL FLOW

Script your ideal day:

_____

_____

_____

_____

_____

_____

_____

4. NIGHTTIME REFLECTION

Improvements   **Successes**

1. _____   1. _____

2. _____   2. _____

3. _____   3. _____

When did you feel in flow today?

_____

_____

1. MORNING GRATEFUL FLOW

What are you grateful for today?

1. _____

2. _____

3. _____

2. FORWARD FOCUS

High-Value Priorities

1. _____

2. _____

3. _____

High-Flow Priorities

1. _____

2. _____

3. _____

Daily Schedule

MORNING: _____

_____

AFTERNOON: _____

_____

NIGHT: _____

3. TOTAL FLOW

Script your ideal day:

_____

_____

_____

_____

_____

_____

_____

4. NIGHTTIME REFLECTION

Improvements   **Successes**

1. _____   1. _____

2. _____   2. _____

3. _____   3. _____

When did you feel in flow today?

_____

_____

I. MORNING GRATEFUL FLOW

What are you grateful for today?

1. _____

2. _____

3. _____

2. FORWARD FOCUS

High-Value Priorities

1. _____

2. _____

3. _____

High-Flow Priorities

1. _____

2. _____

3. _____

Daily Schedule

MORNING: _____

_____

AFTERNOON: _____

_____

NIGHT: _____

_____

3. TOTAL FLOW

Script your ideal day:

_____

_____

_____

_____

_____

_____

_____

4. NIGHTTIME REFLECTION

Improvements   **Successes**

1. _____   1. _____

2. _____   2. _____

3. _____   3. _____

When did you feel in flow today?

_____

_____

NOTES

Preface

1. Mihaly Csikszentmihalyi, "Flow, the Secret to Happiness," TED2004, February 2004, https://www.ted.com/talks/mihaly_csikszentmihalyi_on_flow?utm_campaign=tedspread&utm_medium=referral&utm_source=tedcomshare

Introduction

2. Mihaly Csikszentmihalyi, *Finding Flow: The Psychology of Engagement with Everyday Life* (New York: Basic Books, 1997), 31.
3. Mihaly Csikszentmihalyi, *Flow: The Psychology of Optimal Experience* (New York: Harper & Row, 1990), 217.
4. Ibid., 214.

Morning Grateful Flow

5. Nancy P. Rothbard, "How Your Morning Mood Effects Your Whole Workday," *Harvard Business Review* online, July 21, 2016, https://hbr.org/2016/07/how-your-morning-mood-affects-your-whole-workday
6. Shawn Achor and Michelle Gielan, "Consuming Negative News Can Make You Less Effective at Work, *Harvard Business Review* online, September 14, 2015, https://hbr.org/2015/09/consuming-negative-news-can-make-you-less-effective-at-work

7.   Alex Korb, PhD, *The Upward Spiral: Using Neuroscience to Reverse the Course of Depression, One Small Change at a Time* (Oakland: New Harbinger Publications, Inc., 2015), 154.

8.   Alex Korb, PhD, "The Grateful Brain: The Neuroscience of Giving Thanks, *Psychology Today* online, November 20, 2012, https://www.psychologytoday.com/intl/blog/prefrontal-nudity/201211/the-grateful-brain

9.   Ibid.

10. Robert A. Emmons and Michael E. McCullough, "Counting Blessings Versus Burdens: An Experimental Investigation of Gratitude and Subjective Well-Being in Daily Life," *Journal of Personality and Social Psychology*, 84:2 (2003), 377–89.

11. Summer Allen, PhD, "The Science of Gratitude," A White Paper Prepared for the John Templeton Foundation by the Greater Good Science Center at UC Berkeley," May 2018, https://ggsc.berkeley.edu/images/uploads/GGSC-JTF_White_Paper-Gratitude-FINAL.pdf

12. Sara B. Algoe, Shelly L. Gable, and Natalya C. Maisel, "It's the Little Things: Everyday Gratitude as a Booster Shot for Romantic Relationships," *Personal Relationships*, 17 (2010), 217–33.

13. Lea Waters, "Predicting Job Satisfaction: Contributions of Individual Gratitude and Institutionalized Gratitude," *Psychology*, 3:12A (2012), 1174–76.

14. Adam M. Grant and Amy Wrzesniewski, "I Won't Let You Down . . . or Will I? Core Self-Evaluations, Other-Orientation, Anticipated Guilt and Gratitude, and Job Performance," *Journal of Applied Psychology*, 95:1 (2010), 108–21.

15. Mihaly Csikszentmihalyi, *Finding Flow: The Psychology of Engagement with Everyday Life* (New York: Basic Books, 1997), 22.

16. Alice M. Isen, Kimberly A. Daubman, and Gary P. Nowicki, "Positive Affect Facilitates Creative Problem Solving," *Journal of Personality and Social Psychology*, 52:6 (1987), 1122–31.

17. Alice M. Isen and Kimberly A. Daubman, "The Influence of Affect on Categorization," *Journal of Personality and Social Psychology*, 47:6 (1984), 1206–17.

18. Alice M. Isen and Barbara Means, "The Influence of Positive Affect on Decision-Making Strategy," *Social Cognition*, 2:1 (1983), 18–31.

19. Barbara L. Fredrickson and Christine Branigan, "Positive Emotions Broaden the Scope of Attention and Thought-Action Repertoires," *Cognition and Emotion*, 19:3 (2005), 313–32.

20. Alex M. Wood, Stephen Joseph, and Alex P. Linley, "Coping Style as a Psychological Resource of Grateful People," *Journal of Social and Clinical Psychology*, 26:9 (2007), 1076–93.

Forward Focus

21. Tim Kreider, "The 'Busy' Trap," *The New York Times* online, June 30,2012, https://opinionator.blogs.nytimes.com/2012/06/30/the-busy-trap/

22. Ibid.

23. Brené Brown, Daring Greatly: How to Courage to Be Vulnerable Transforms the Way We Live, Love, Parent, and Lead (New York: Gotham Books, 2012), 137.

24. Elizabeth Evitts Dickinson, "The Cult of Busy," Johns Hopkins Health Review, 3:1 (2016), 26–37.

25. Robert A. Emmons, "Personal Goals, Life Meaning, and Virtue: Wellsprings of a Positive Life," in Corey L. M. Keyes and Jonathan Haidt (eds.), *Flourishing: Positive Psychology and the Life Well-Lived* (Washington DC: American Psychological Association, 2003), 109.

26. Ibid.

27. Mihaly Csikszentmihalyi, *Finding Flow: The Psychology of Engagement with Everyday Life* (New York: Basic Books, 1997), 34.

28. Cassie Mogilner, "The Pursuit of Happiness: Time, Money, and Social Connection," *Psychological Science*, 21:9 (2010), 1348–54.

29. American Psychological Association, "Multitasking: Switching Costs," *American Psychological Association* website, March 20, 2006, https://www.apa.org/research/action/multitask

30. William R. Klemm, PhD, "The Perils of Multitasking: Your Smart Phone Can Make You Dumb," *Psychology Today* online, August 26, 2016, https://www.psychologytoday.com/gb/blog/memory-medic/201608/the-perils-multitasking

31. Jennifer Robinson, "Too Many Interruptions at Work? Office Distractions Are Worse Than You Think—and Maybe Better," *Gallup* website, June 8, 2006, https://news.gallup.com/businessjournal/23146/too-many-interruptions-work.aspx#1)

Total Flow

32. Tristan Harris, "How a Handful of Tech Companies Control Billions of Minds Every Day," *TED2017*, April 2017, https://www.ted.com/talks/tristan_harris_the_manipulative_tricks_tech_companies_use_to_capture_your_attention/transcript

33. Ibid.

34. Paul Greenberg, "In Search of Lost Screen Time," *The New York Times* online, December 31, 2018, https://www.nytimes.com/2018/12/31/opinion/smartphones-screen-time.html

35. Liz Fuller-Wright, "The Spotlight of Attention Is More like a Strobe, Say Researchers," Princeton University website, August 22, 2018, https://www.princeton.edu/news/2018/08/22/spotlight-attention-more-strobe-say-researchers

36. "How Much Information Is There in the World," University of Southern California website, February 10, 2011, https://pressroom.usc.edu/how-much-information-is-there-in-the-world/

37. Mihaly Csikszentmihalyi and Isabella Selega Csikszentmihalyi (eds.), *Optimal Experience: Psychological Studies of Flow in Consciousness* (New York: Cambridge University Press, 1988), 18.

38. William James, *The Principles of Psychology, Vol. 1* (New York: Henry Holt and Company, 1890), 402.

39. Liz Fuller-Wright, "The Spotlight of Attention Is More like a Strobe, Say Researchers," Princeton University website, August 22, 2018, https://www.princeton.edu/

news/2018/08/22/spotlight-attention-more-strobe-say-researchers

40. Claire Calmels, Christelle Berthoumieux, and Fabienne D'Arripe-Longueville, "Effects of an Imagery Training Program on Selective Attention of National Softball Players," *The Sport Psychologist*, 18:3 (2004), 272–96.

41. Christopher Clarey, "Olympians Use Imagery as Mental Training, *The New York Times* online, February 22, 2014, https://www.nytimes.com/2014/02/23/sports/olympics/olympians-use-imagery-as-mental-training.html

42. Ibid.

43. Adam R. Nicholls, Remco C.J. Polman, and Nicholas L. Holt, "The Effects of an Individualized Imagery Interventions on Flow States and Golf Performance," Athletic Insight, 7:1 (2005), 43–66.

44. Krista J. Munroe-Chandler and Michelle D. Guerrero, "Psychological Imagery in Sport and Performance," *Oxford Research Encyclopedia of Psychology* online, 2017, https://oxfordre.com/psychology/view/10.1093/acrefore/9780190236557.001.0001/acrefore-9780190236557-e-228

Nighttime Reflection

45. Timothy D. Wilson, David A. Reinhard, Erin C. Westgate, Daniel T. Gilbert, Nicole Ellerbeck, Cheryl Hahn, Casey L. Brown, and Adi Shaked, "Just think: The Challenges of the Disengaged Mind," Science, 345:6192 (2014), 75–7.

46. Tasha Eurich, "What Self-Awareness Really Is (and How to Cultivate It), *Harvard Business Review* online, January 4, 2018, https://hbr.org/2018/01/what-self-awareness-really-is-and-how-to-cultivate-it

47. Anna Sutton, Helen M. Williams, and Christopher W. Allinson, "A Longitudinal, Mixed Method Evaluation of Self-Awareness Training in the Workplace," *European Journal of Training and Development*, 39:7 (2015), 610–27.

48. Bernard M. Bass and Francis J. Yammarino, "Congruence of Self and Others' Leadership Ratings of Naval Officers for Understanding Successful Performance," *Applied Psychology*, 40:4 (2008), 437–54.

49. Paul J. Silvia and Maureen E. O'Brien, "Self-Awareness and Constructive Functioning: Revisiting 'the Human Dilemma,' " *Journal of Social and Clinical Psychology*, 23:4 (2004), 475–89.

50. Michael K. Scullin, Madison L. Krueger, Hannah K. Ballard, Natalya Pruett, and Donal L. Bliwise, "The Effects of Bedtime Writing on Difficulty Falling Asleep: A Polysomnographic Study Comparing To-Do Lists and Completed Activity Lists," *Journal of Experimental Psychology: General*, 147:1 (2018), 139–46.

51. Lydia Denworth, "The Connection between Writing and Sleeping," *Psychology Today* online, January 12, 2018, https://www.psychologytoday.com/us/blog/brain-waves/201801/the-connection-between-writing-and-sleep

52. Ethan Kross, Emma Bruehlman-Senecal, Jiyoung Park, Aleah Burson, Adrienne Dougherty, Holly Shablack, Ryan Bremner, Jason Moser, and Ozlem Ayduk, "Self-Talk as a Regulatory Mechanism: How You do It Matters," *Journal of Personality and Social Psychology*, 106:2 (2014), 304–24.

53. Ethan Kross and Ozlem Ayduk, "Making Meaning out of Negative Experiences by Self-Distancing," *Current Directions in Psychological Science*, 20:3 (2011), 187–91.

54. Kate Murphy, "No Time to Think," *The New York Times* online, July 25, 2014, https://www.nytimes.com/2014/07/27/sunday-review/no-time-to-think.html

55. Tasha Eurich, "What Self-Awareness Really Is (and How to Cultivate It), *Harvard Business Review* online, January 4, 2018, https://hbr.org/2018/01/what-self-awareness-really-is-and-how-to-cultivate-it

56. Mihaly Csikszentmihalyi, *Finding Flow: The Psychology of Engagement with Everyday Life* (New York: Basic Books, 1997), 47.

INDEX

ACKNOWLEDGMENTS

I would like to thank my husband, Chris. I am truly grateful for your unwavering belief, love, and support.

Thank you to my inspiring brother, Daniel, talented sister, Eve, and the O'Rawe and the Gregg families—your unshakable support helped me write this book. I would also like to thank my Mum for helping to shape the person that I am today.

A special thank you to all my friends thanks for always having my back, listening without judgment, and making me laugh.

And finally, a huge thank you to my publisher, Rage Kindelsperger and editor, Erin Canning, without whom this book would not have been possible. A heartfelt thank you for seeing my potential, for all your expertise and guidance, and for making my childhood dream of becoming a writer come true.

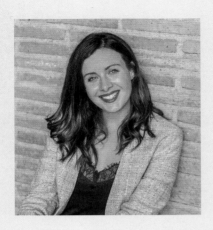

ABOUT THE AUTHOR

SARAH GREGG is a Northern Irish girl with a huge passion for unlocking human potential (you could call it a bit of an obsession). She is a member of the British Psychological Society, a certified life coach, a business coach, and a certified neurolinguistic programming practitioner. Sarah prides herself on her professional advice and coaching. She has had a diverse career, during which she has worked with hundreds of individuals and businesses, big and small—from large corporate clients to start-ups and entrepreneurs. The common thread that runs throughout her career is her passion for helping people realize their potential. At the end of 2016, she took a bold leap into the unknown. Practicing what she preaches, she went after her own goals and established The Power to Reinvent (www.thepowertoreinvent.com). You can connect with her on Instagram @powertoreinvent.

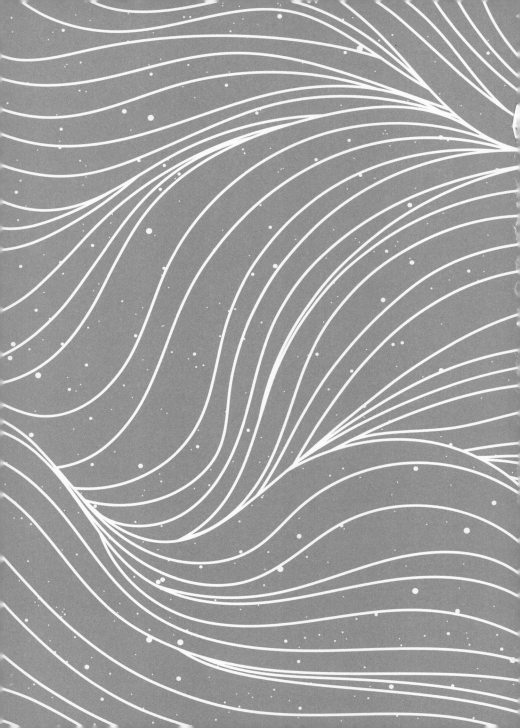